Why Can't I Pay Attention

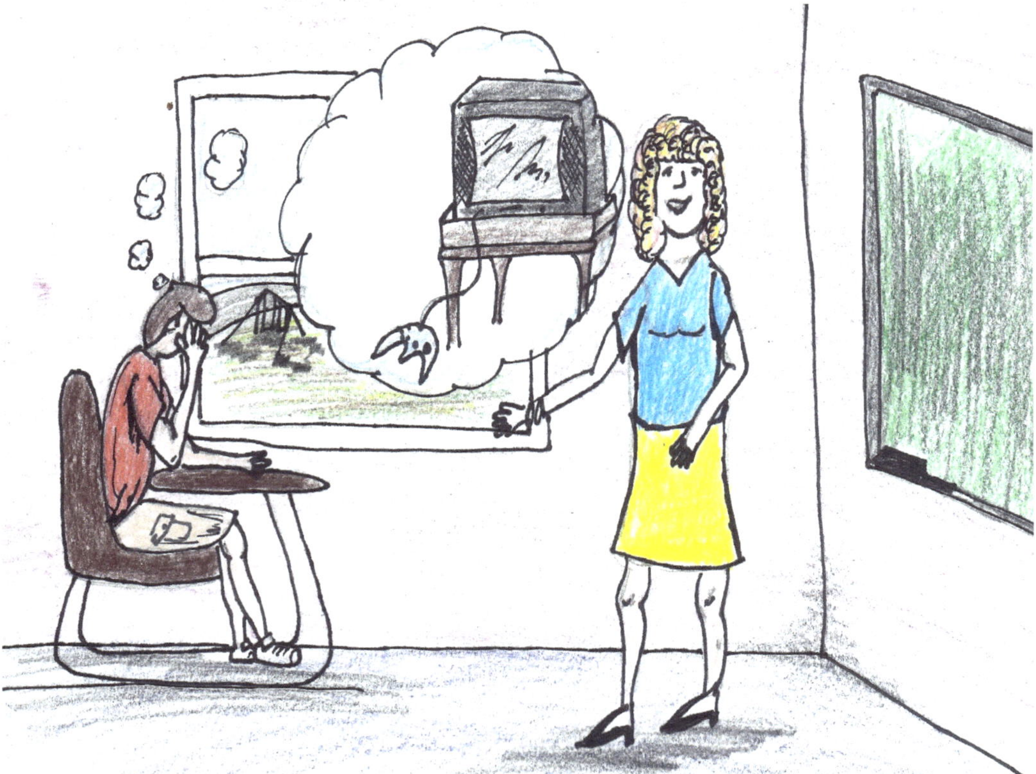

By

Lynn Dickerson

Illustrated by Faith East

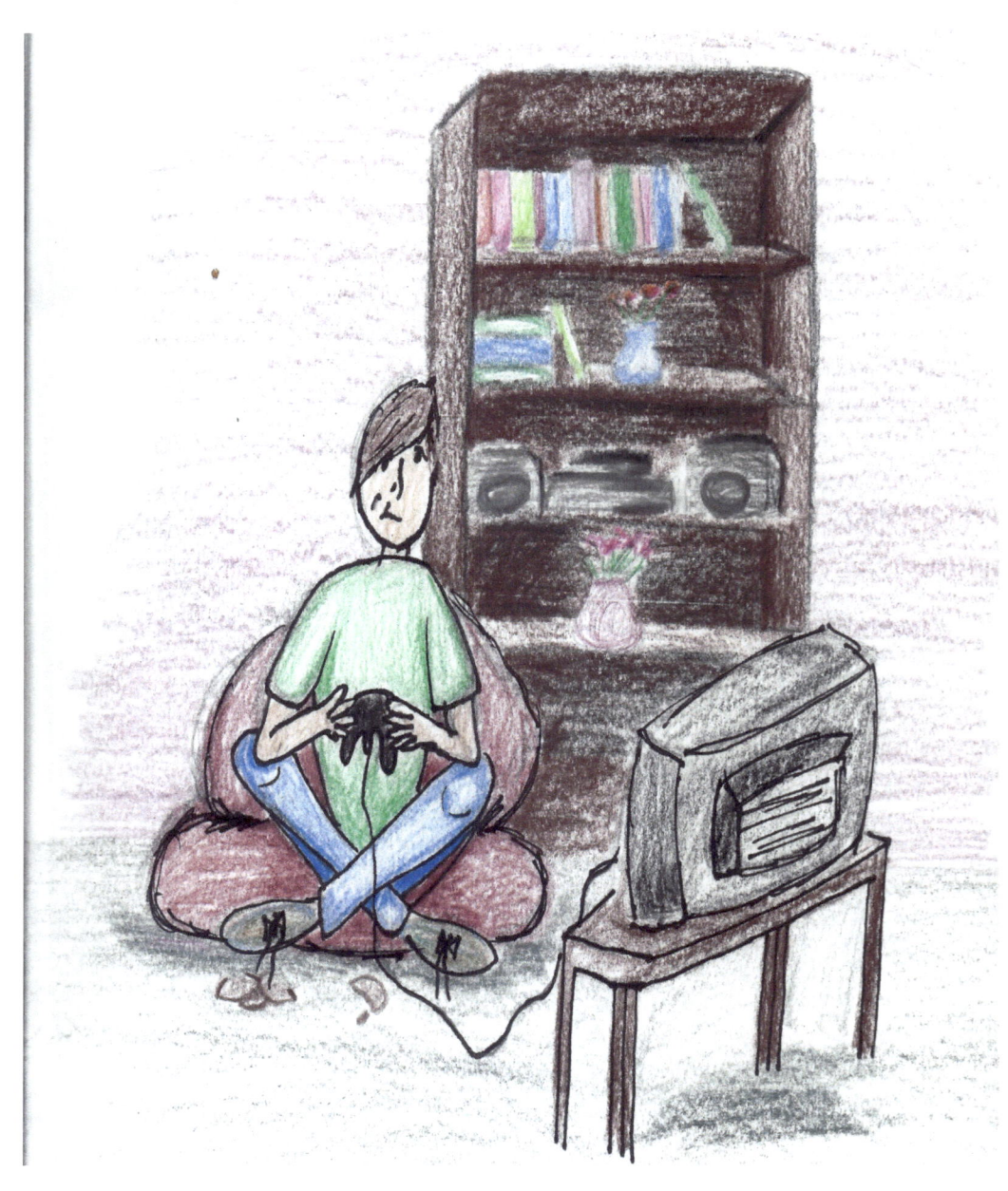

ISBN 149098545X

ISBN-13:978-1490985459

ACKNOWLEDGMENTS

I Appreciate the encouragement from friends and family who recognized children needed a book like this. Thank you David, Sarah, Randy and Cindy

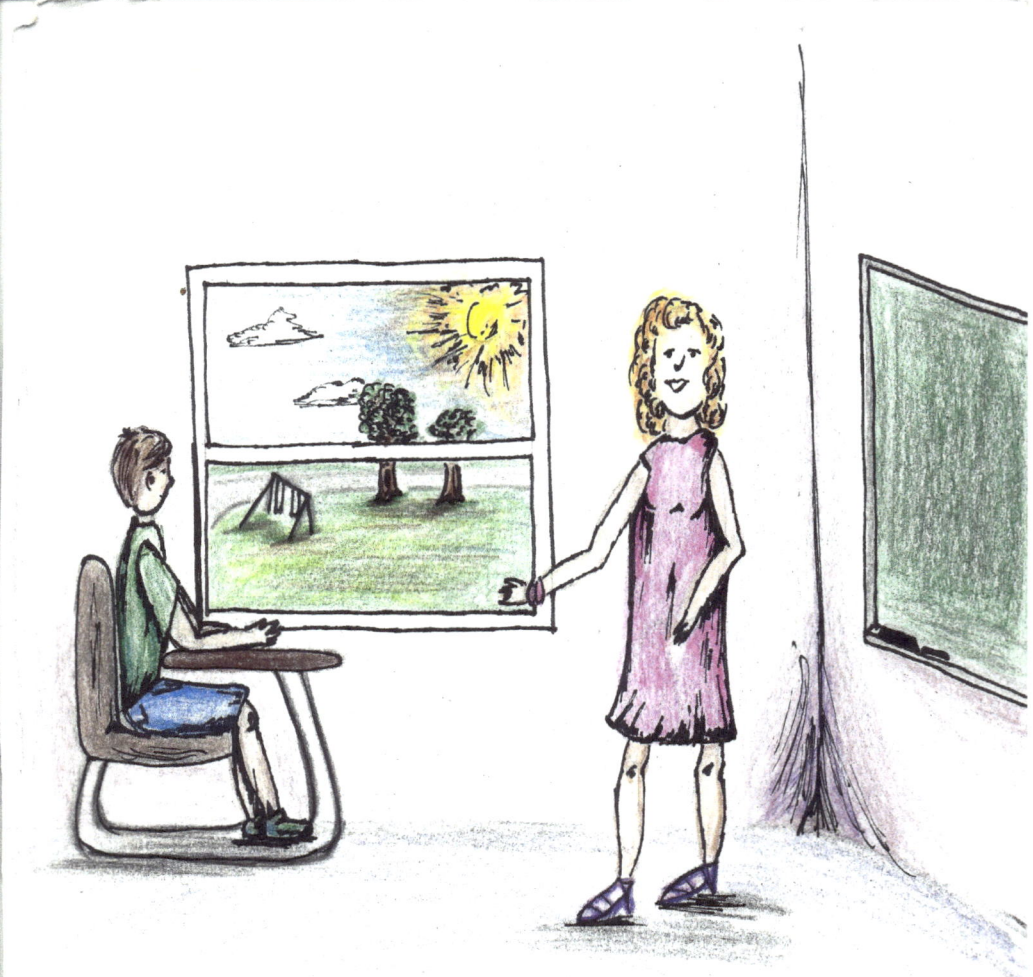

A boy named Paul was sitting in his fourth grade class. The day was warm and sunny. The wind was blowing and the flowers were starting to bud with all their different colors. The sun was shining so bright you could almost feel it shining on your skin just by looking out the window. "I could probably kick a soccer ball between those two trees", thought Paul.

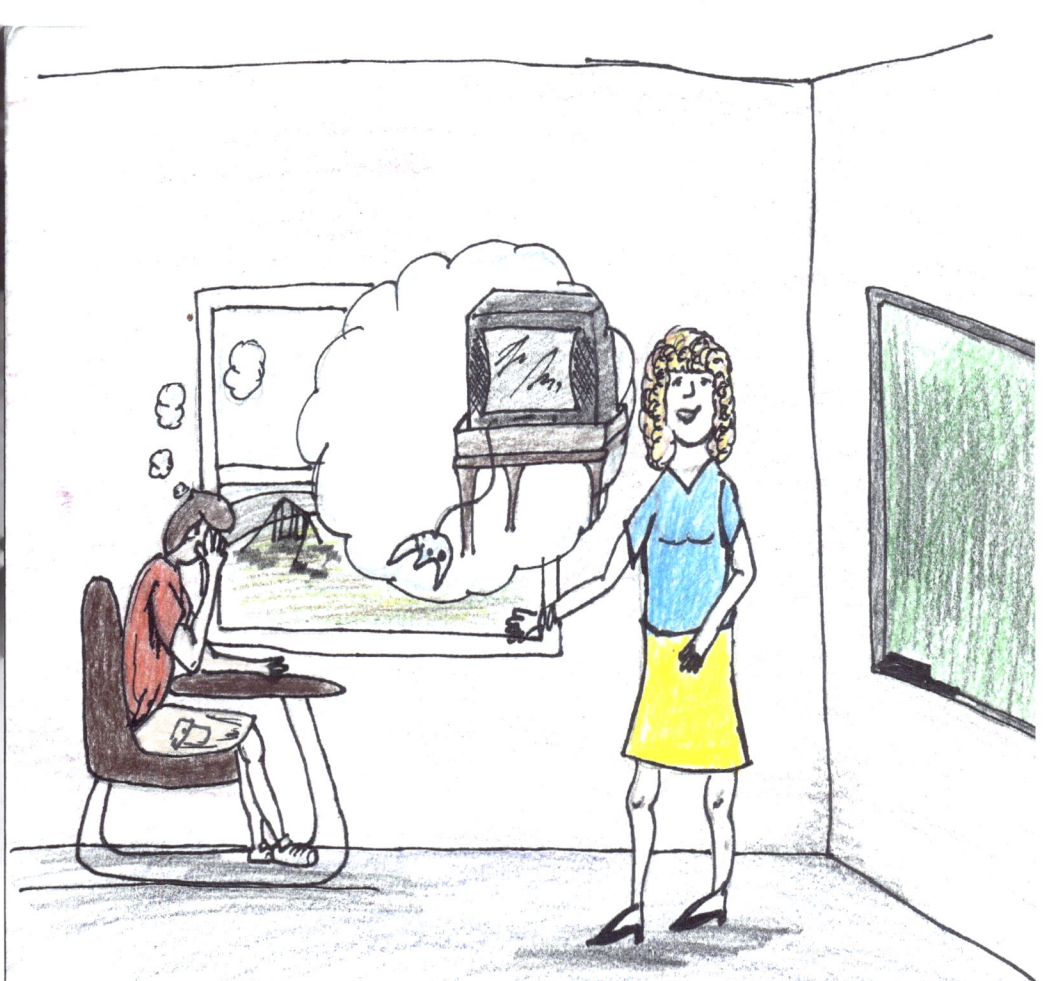

Just then Mrs. Smith asked Paul to name the states that border the Great Lakes; she has talked about these states for the last thirty minutes. Now Paul realized he was looking out the window and had no idea what the teacher was talking about. Paul looked at the teacher and thought "why can't I pay attention. I like Mrs. Smith and I want to make good grades but I can't keep my mind on what is going on in the class room."

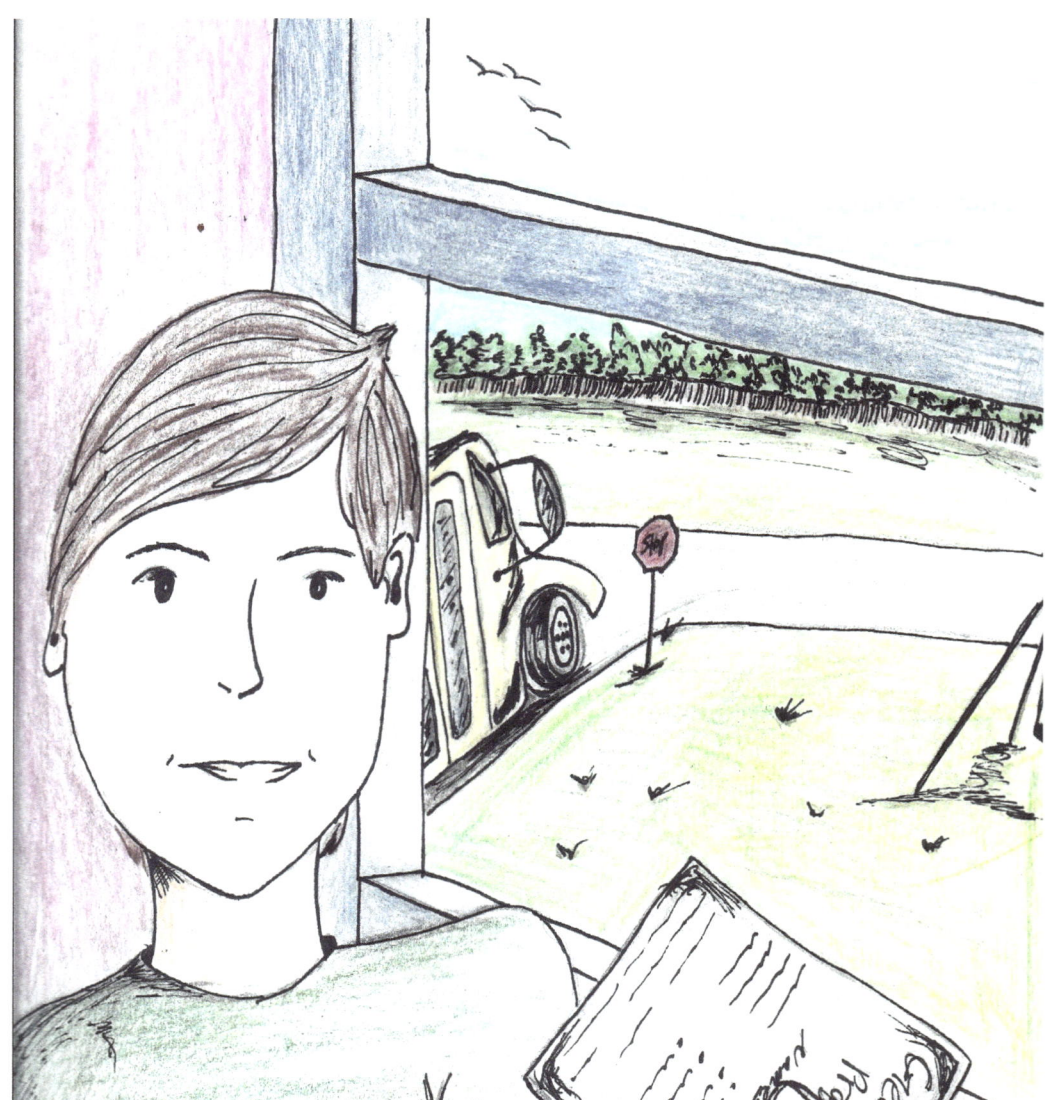

Seems he never remembers what someone says, if they talk too long. Paul did that a lot. If Mom tells him to do something he will never remembers until Mom brings it up again.

Before the class leaves Mrs. Smith's room for the day she tells the class about their geography project due next Friday. It is Friday so Paul says to himself "Good I have a week to do the project".

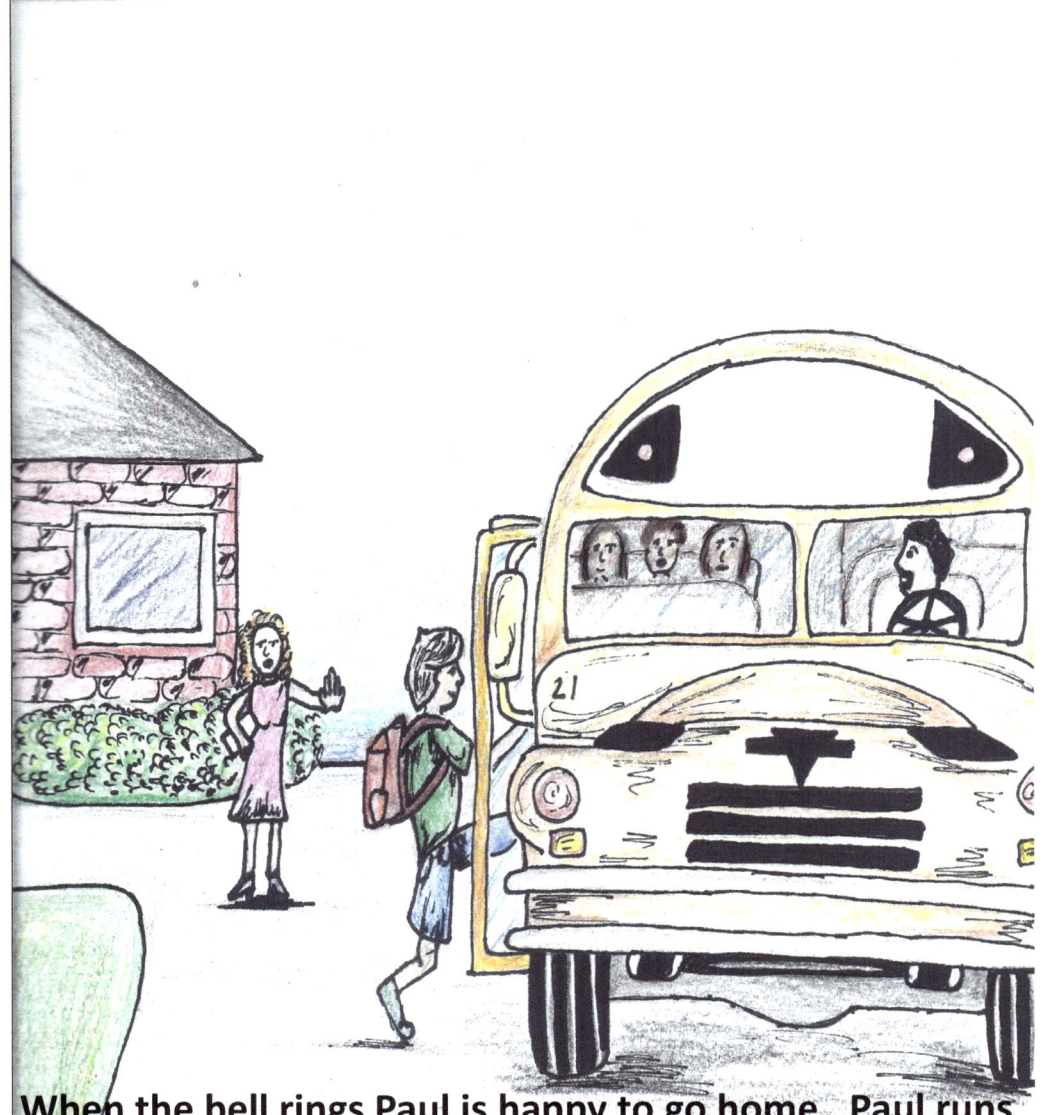

When the bell rings Paul is happy to go home. Paul runs to the bus even though a teacher is telling him to stop running. But what she says never registers in Paul's mind. When he gets to the bus the bus driver tells him gruffly, "that teacher told you to stop running three times". "Not again" Paul thinks, "I get in trouble all the time for things I never hear. Everybody just likes to fuss at me".

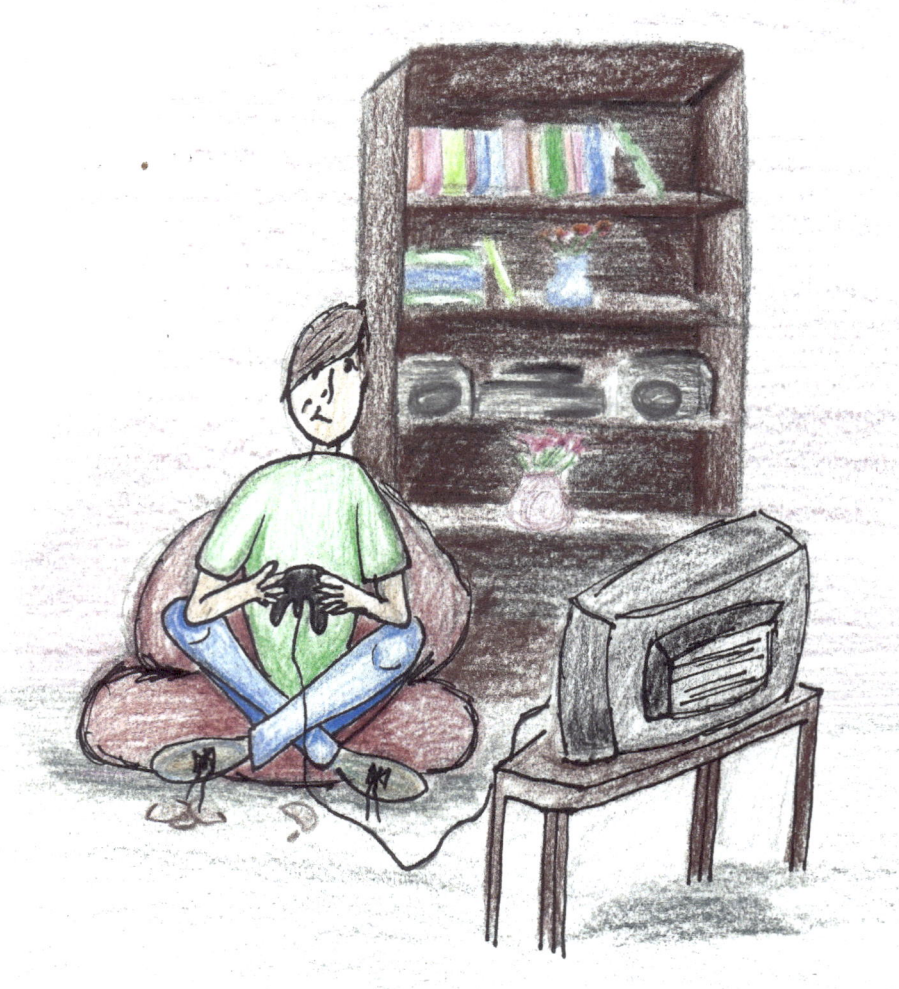

When Paul gets home he can't wait to play his new video game, Bulldog Run. He runs in the house, drops his book bag just inside the door, runs to the kitchen, and grabs a hand full of cookies. He runs to his room, grabs his game and begins to play his new game.

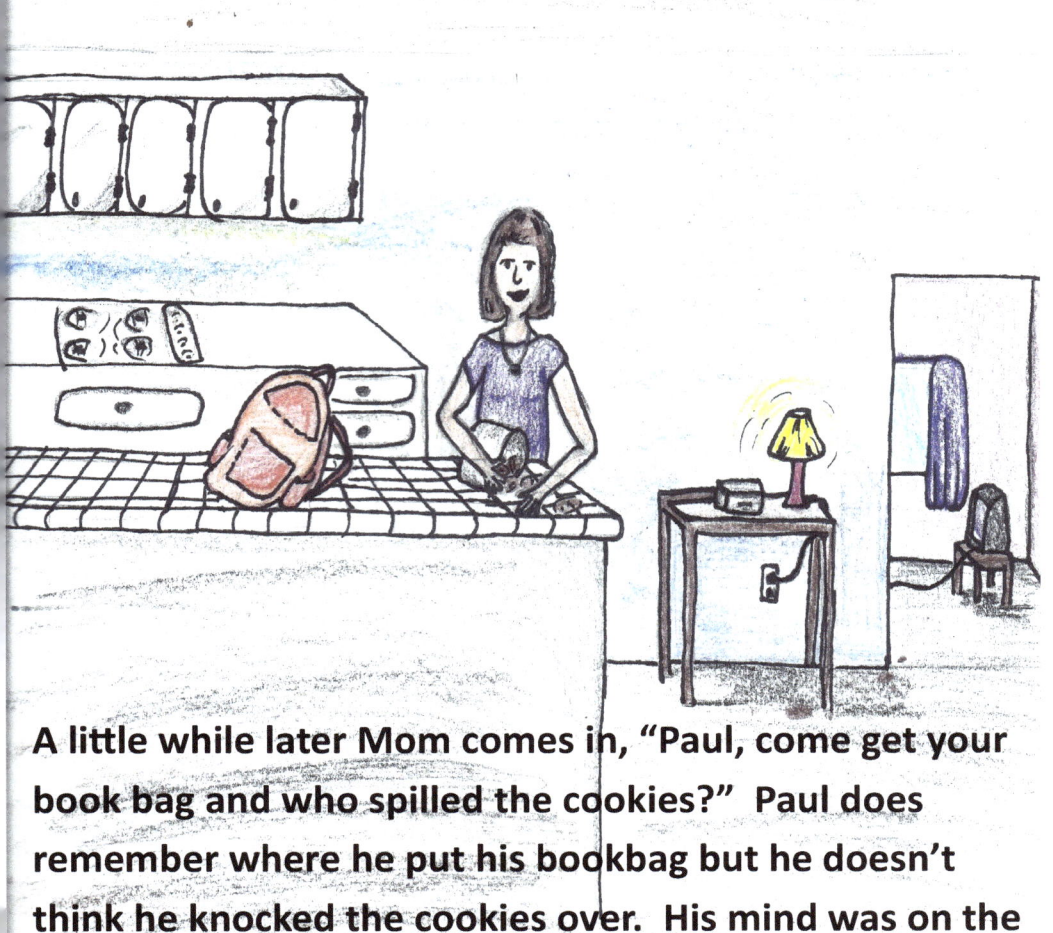

A little while later Mom comes in, "Paul, come get your book bag and who spilled the cookies?" Paul does remember where he put his bookbag but he doesn't think he knocked the cookies over. His mind was on the game. Later Mom comes into his room," Paul come pick up your book bag. I told you to come get it an hour ago. Also come pick the cookies up you spilled". "I didn't spill the cookies Mom" Paul said. Mom said back in frustration "Paul who else would spill them, no one else was in the house." Paul thinks, "Why do I always get into trouble. I hate always getting into trouble".

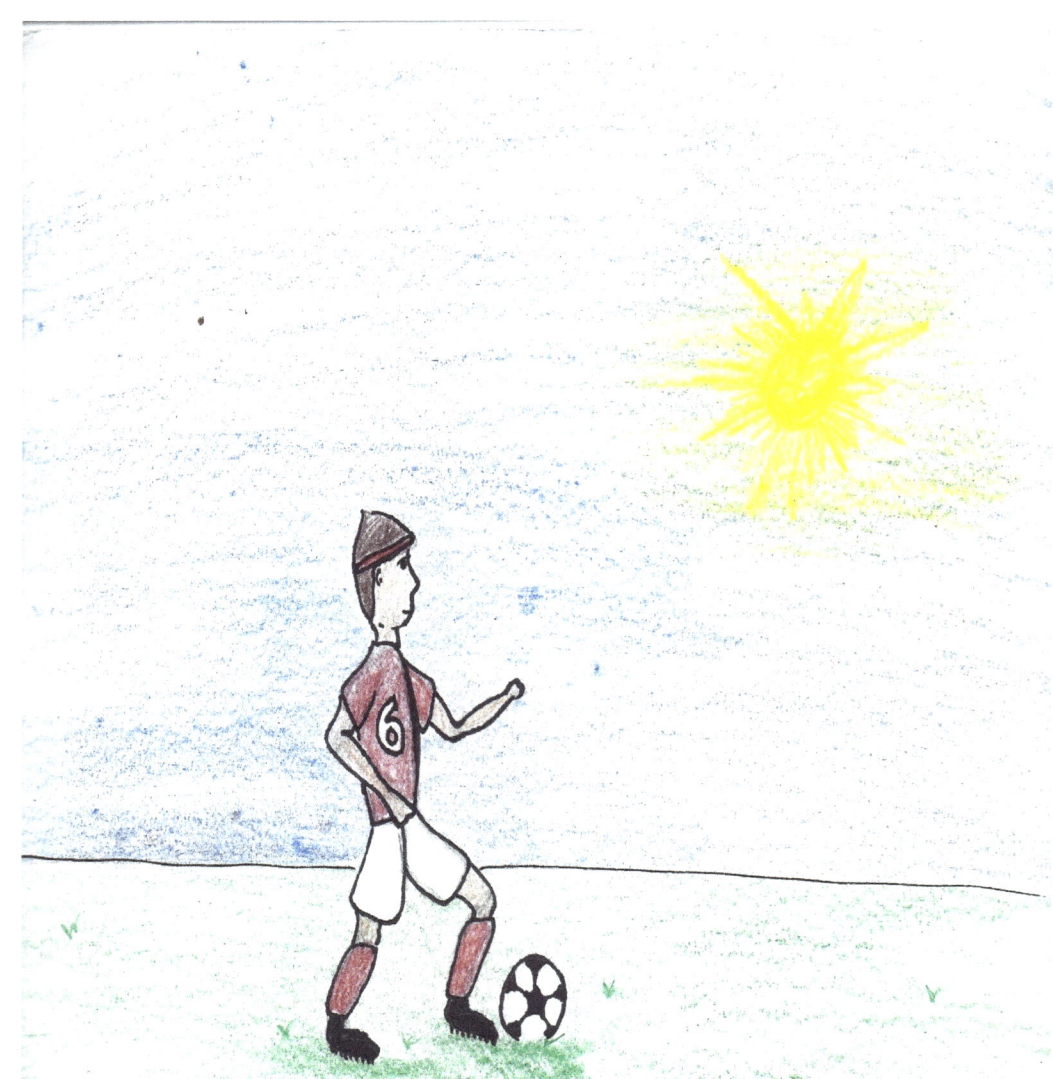

The weekend went as normal in a blur, full of Soccer games and baseball practice. Paul can concentrate when he does things he can move around doing. In fact Paul finds if he does not have things to do physically he finds himself playing with what ever is close. Mom is always fussing at him about what she calls fidgeting. He will pick up something to play with and never remember where he put what he had in his hand.

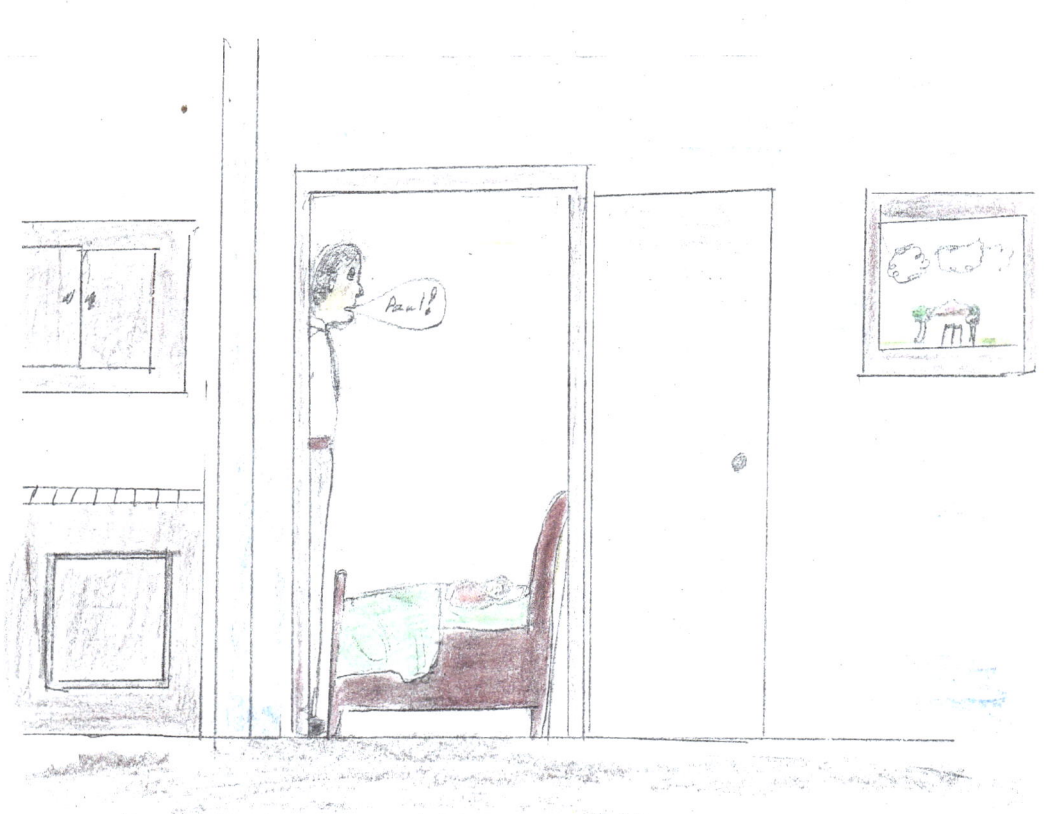

When Monday comes around Paul grabs his book bag
after getting dressed and had to hurry. He got up late
even though Dad told him to get up three times. Paul
never heard him until the third time when Dad was
really mad after telling him to get up three times.

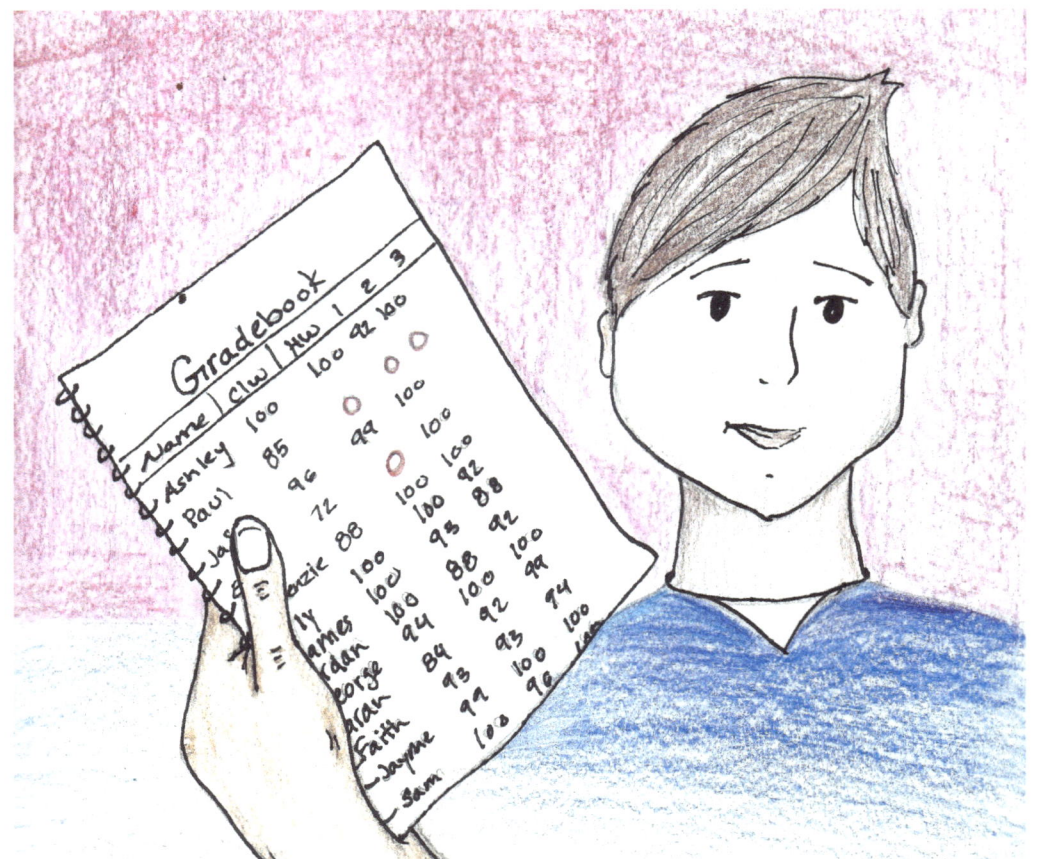

When Paul gets to school Monday the first thing the teacher says is to get their home work out. "Oh no, I forgot" thought Paul. When the teacher comes by to check his work, Paul tries to explain to the teacher he was too busy this weekend to get his homework but it didn't work. Paul really knew he also watched a lot of TV when he could have done his homework but it never crossed his mind. This was the third zero he has gotten this term. Mom and Dad are really going to be mad now. "Why do I keep forgetting? I want to do well in school. It makes Mom so happy when I do well. It is just so hard to remember everything I need to do." .

Report Card

Students Name: Paul

Subject:	Grade:	Letter Grade:
Math	71	C
English	65	D
Social studies	68	D
Spel...	58	F
S...e	70	C

The end of the term comes around and Paul's grades look like:

Math 71

English 65

Social Studies 68

Spelling 58

9

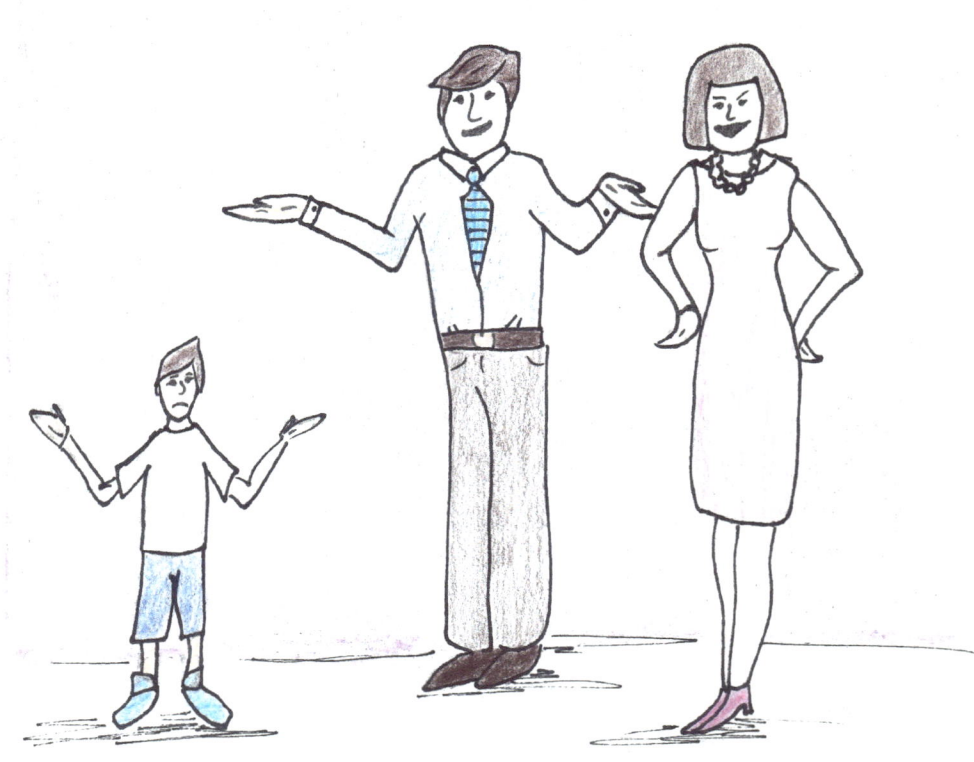

Mom and Dad are upset at Paul for making such low grades. They know he has the ability to make better grades. Paul tries to give reasons like; "I didn't get a copy of the work and the teacher would not give me one or someone stole my work," even though Paul knew he really lost it and forgot the other. Paul's excuses seem to work less and less on his parents.

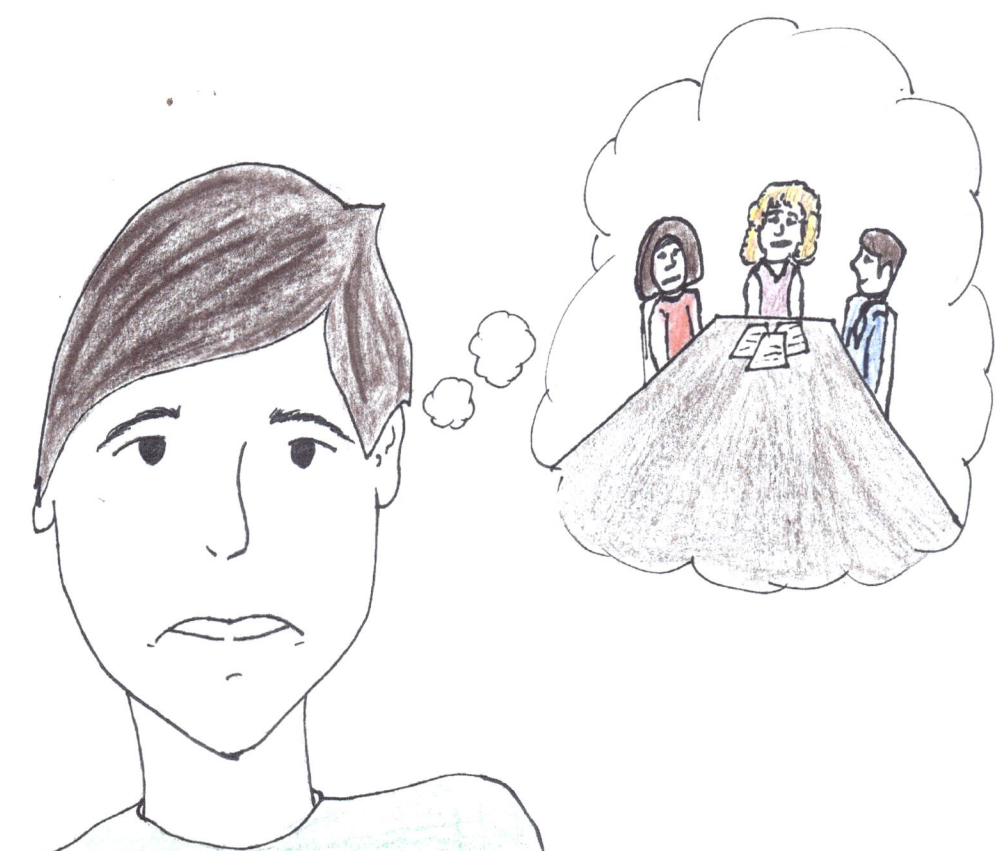

Paul's Parents set a meeting with his teachers. Paul could not think about anything else that day. His mind was on the meeting. That afternoon when Paul's parents came to pick him up after school, they discussed with him what the teachers said. All his teachers talked about how smart he was but he did not turn in work and was easily distracted while attempting his work. His organization needed help and he needed to try harder at finishing his work and projects.

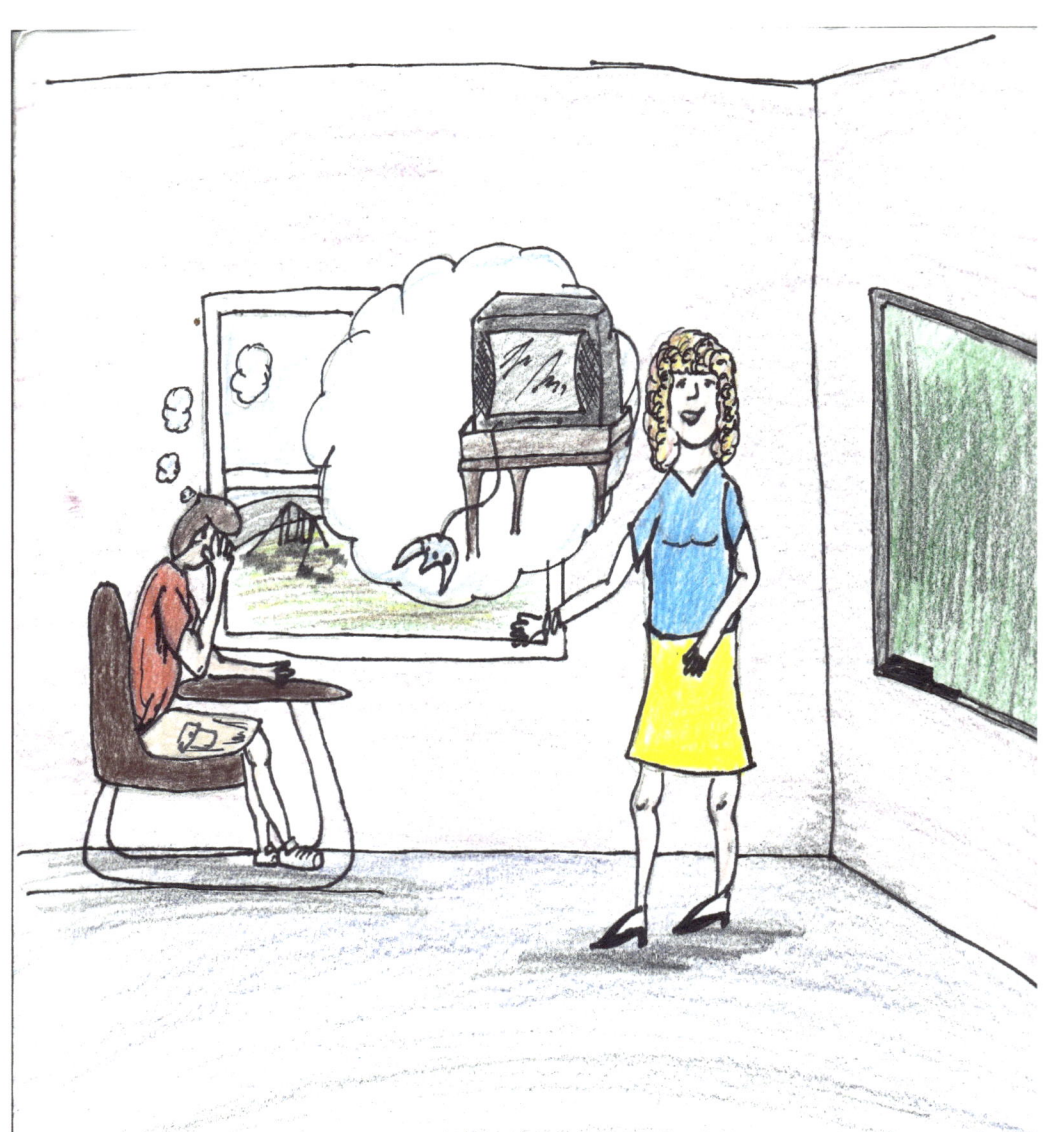

This was not new things coming from his teachers.
Teachers in years past said the same things. But Paul
did try and tried hard. He just had a hard time
keeping his mind on what he should. His brain just
seems to run away sometimes.

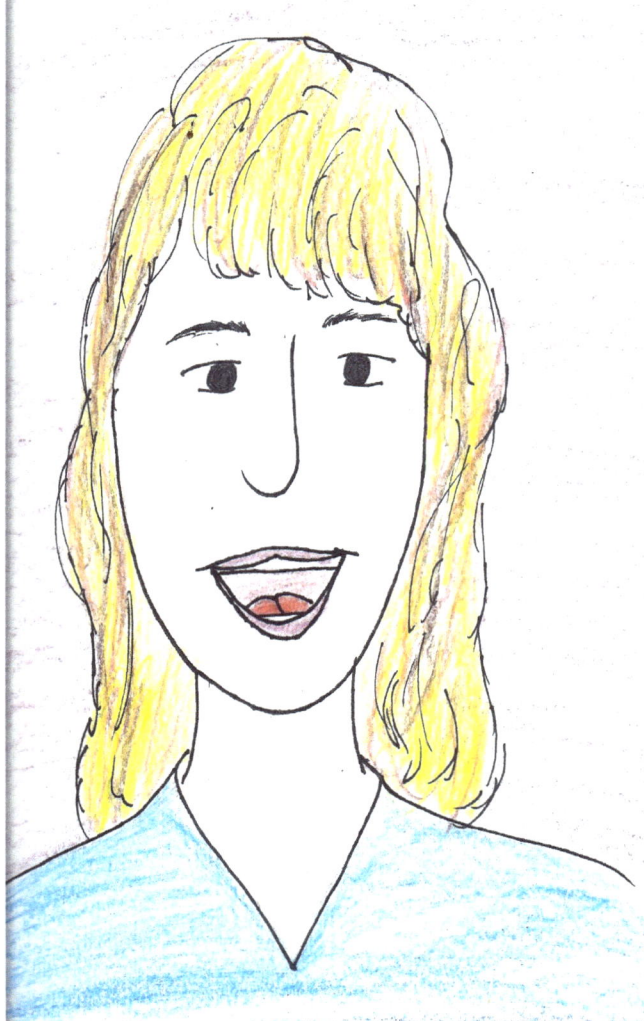

One of Paul's teachers asked if he had been tested for ADD. Paul's first thoughts were; "I don't want to be tested for some kind of disease. What would my friends think if I had this disease. Will the other kids want to play with him?"

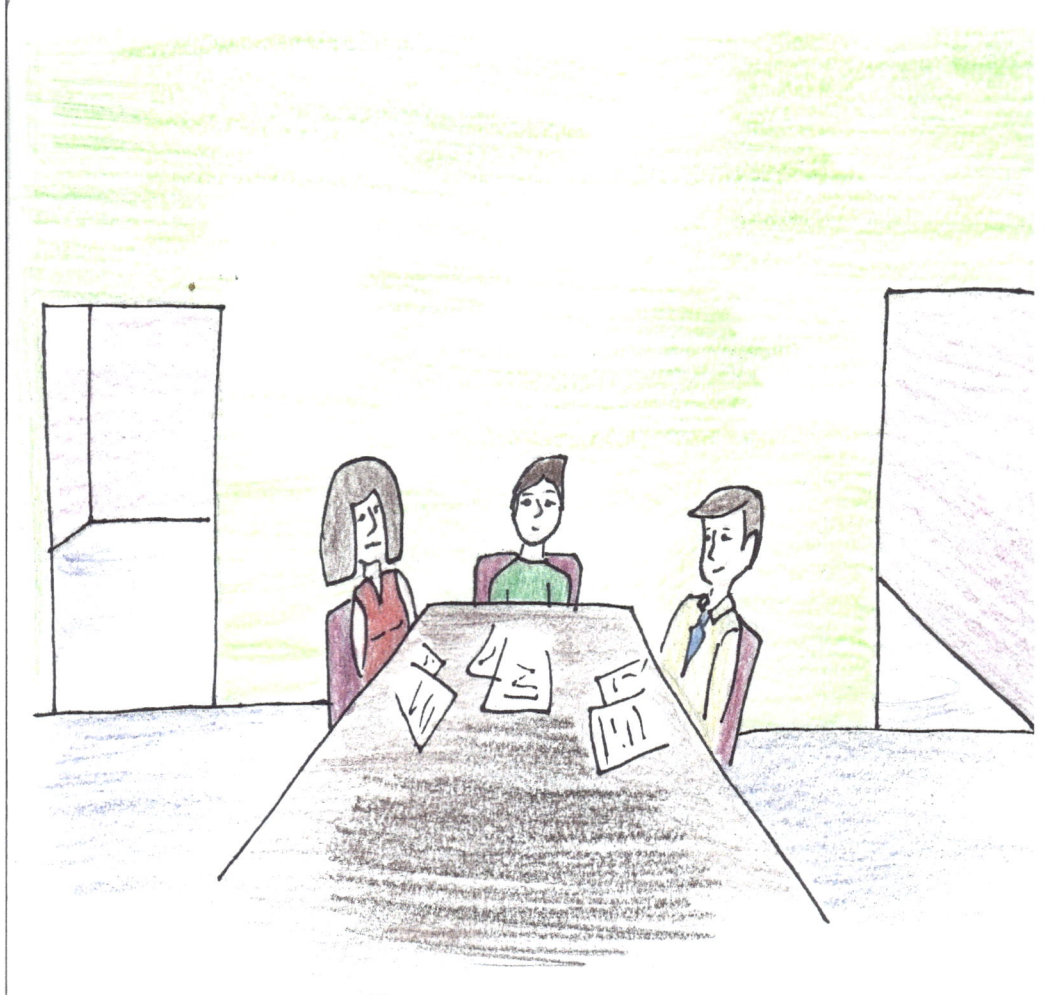

Paul's parents explained that ADD stands for Attention Deficit Disorder and it would not be such a bad thing. It is not a disease and you can't catch it from other people. If he was diagnosed with ADD it would just help them find a way to help Paul with his issues in school, like having a difficult time paying attention in class.

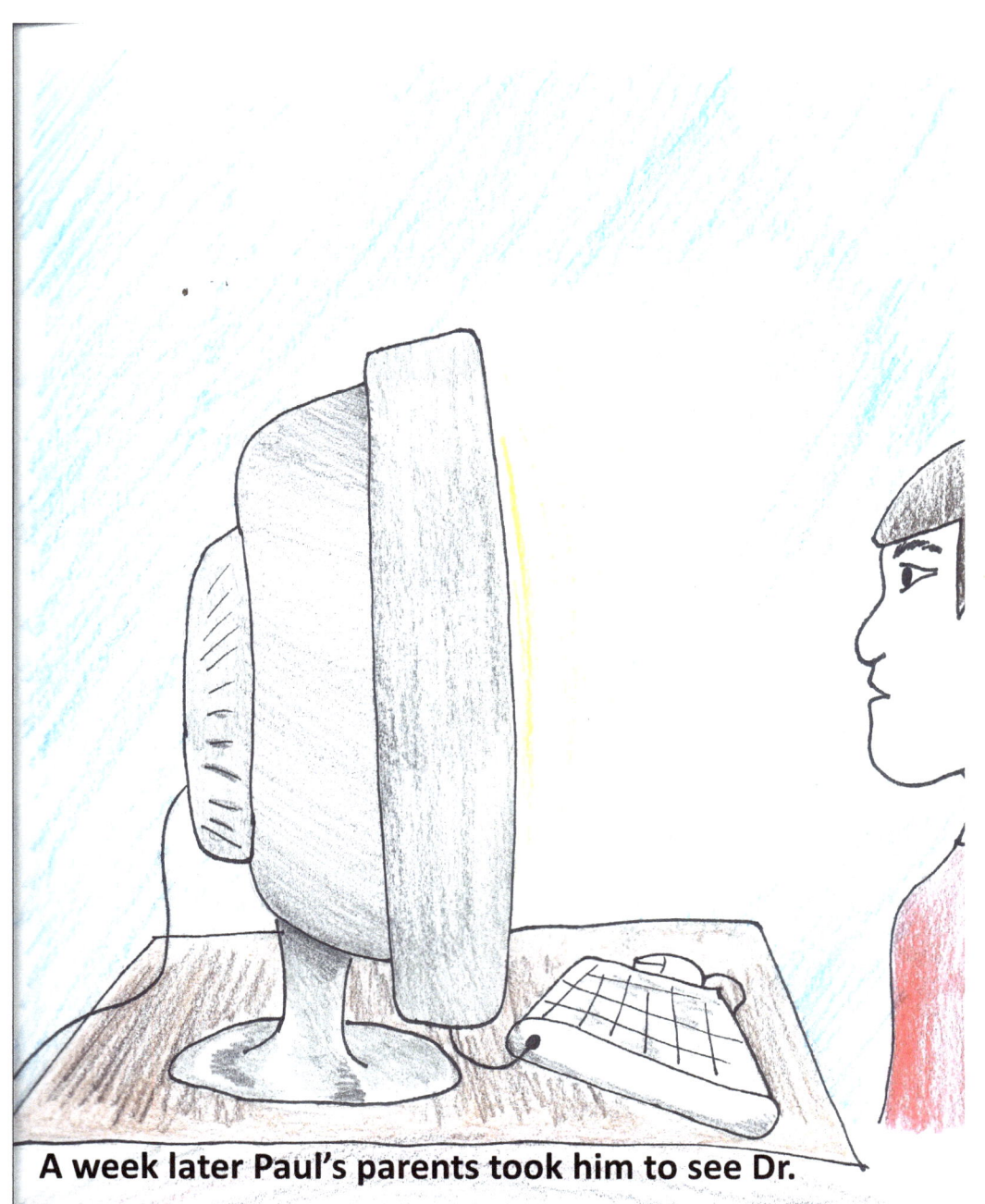

 A week later Paul's parents took him to see Dr.
Williams , a very nice man, he asked Paul some
questions about himself. He also asked Paul to take a
test on the computer. While Paul was taking the test
the doctor asked Paul's parents to fill out a question-
naire about Paul.

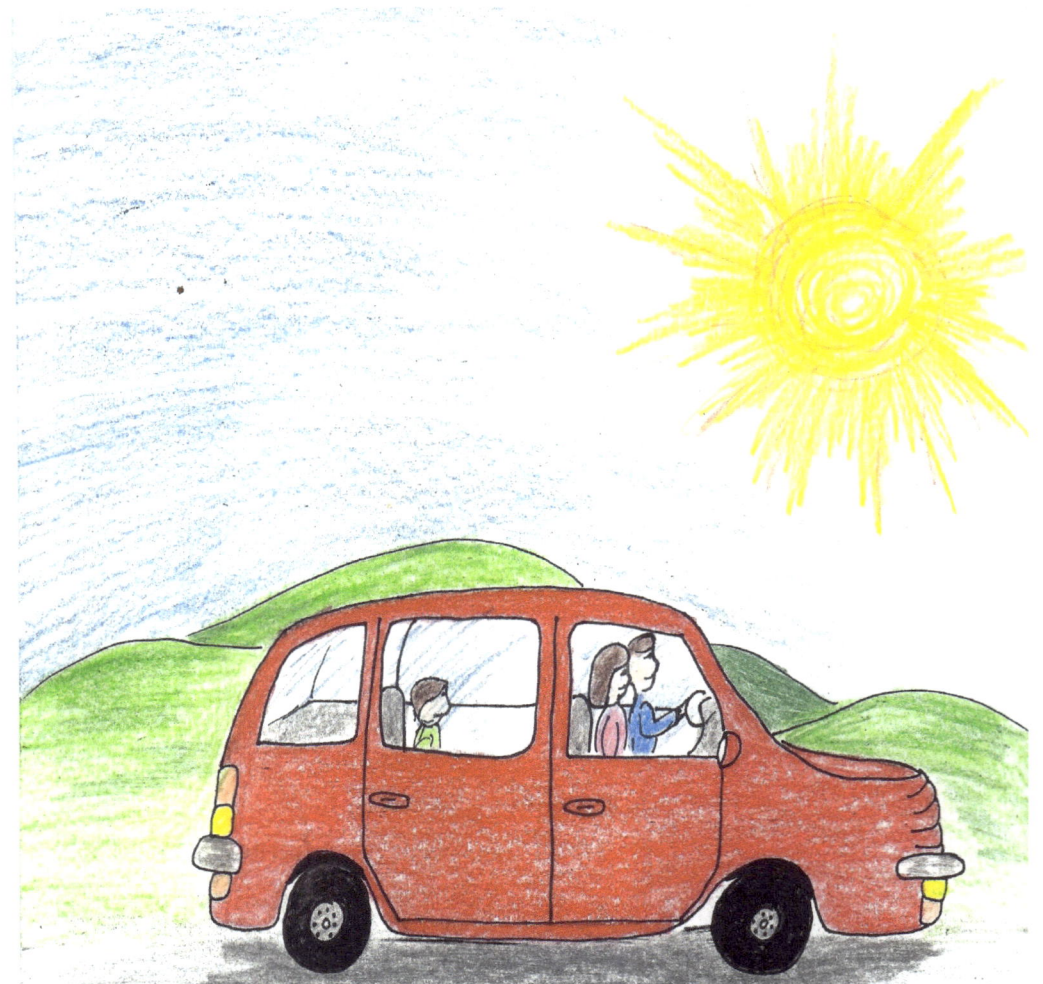

When Paul was finished Dr. Williams talked to Paul's parents and then they left. On the way home, Paul's parents talked to him about what Dr. Williams said. Dr. Williams said that Paul was ADD and Paul was also very intelligent. They said that ADD just means that something in his brain just works different. ADD stands for Attention Deficit Disorder. The doctor gave them some medicine that would help Paul pay attention in class until he learns other ways to manage his ADD.

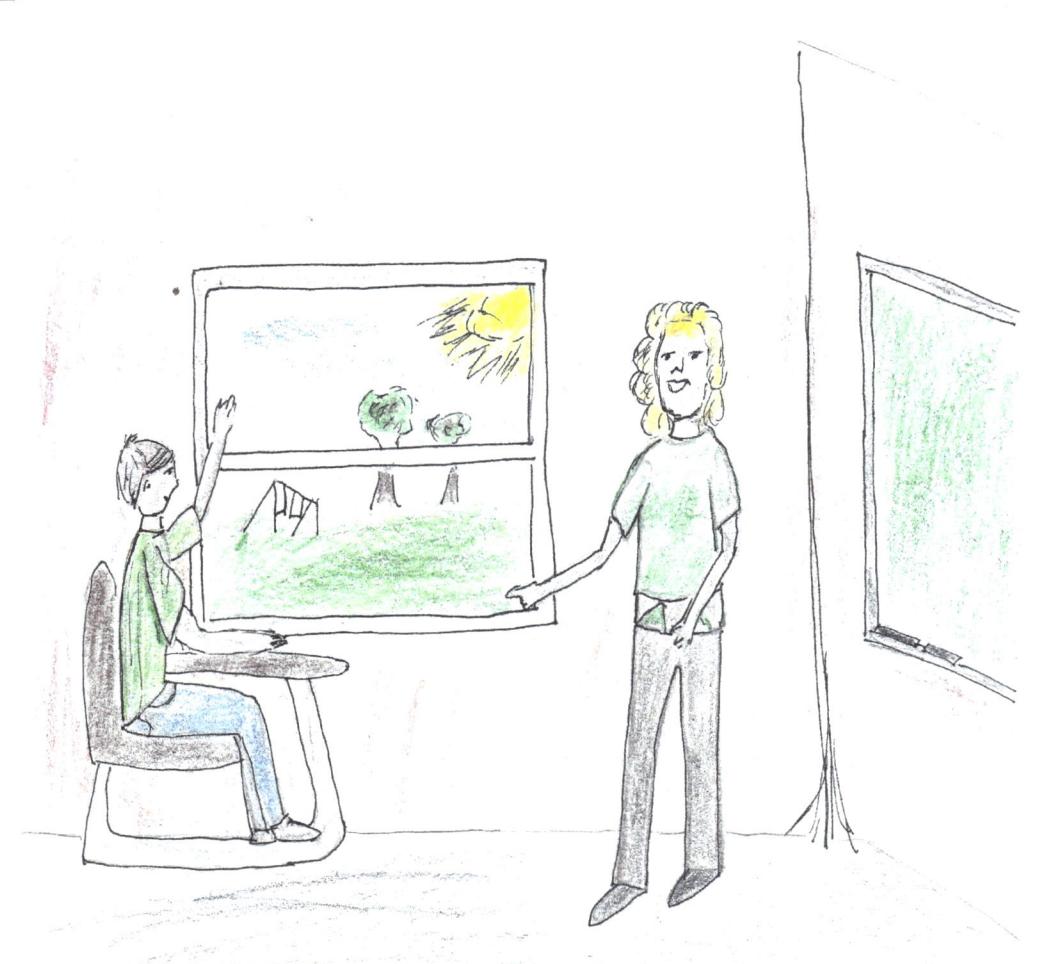

The next week Paul was sitting in his geography class.
His teacher asked a question about the subject she has
been talking about for the last few days. Paul raised his
hand, the teacher calls on him and he gives the correct
answer. "Good Paul, that is correct "said Mrs. Smith.
Paul never answered questions willingly in class and it
sure felt good to do well.

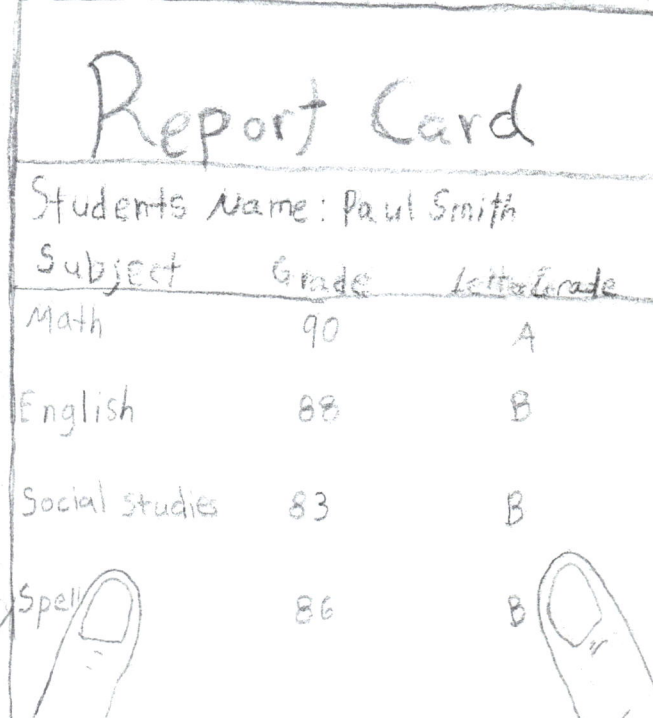

Report Card

Students Name: Paul Smith

Subject	Grade	Letter Grade
Math	90	A
English	88	B
Social studies	83	B
Spelling	86	B

A few weeks later Paul received his second term report card;

Math 90

English 88

Social Studies 85

Spelling 86

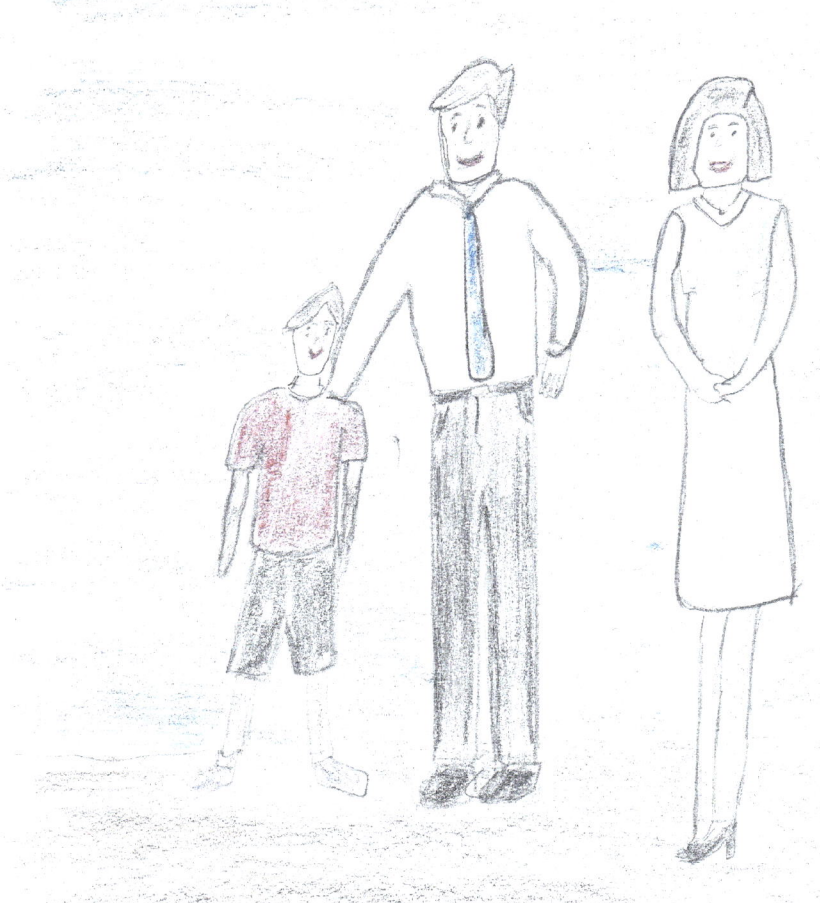

When Paul got home he showed his parents his report card. Both Mom and Dad were very happy. Paul was happy too, his grades were not the best in class but they are a good start. Now Paul knows he can do well and next term he knows he will do even better.

ABOUT THE AUTHOR

Lynn Dickerson has worked in education for thirty three years, twenty five years in the classroom and eight years as a guidance counselor. She has taught many ADD/ADHD children and saw the frustration they went through trying to be successful in school. Raising a son with ADHD as well as having taught many children with ADD/ADHD inspired her to research ways to help these children to be successful in the classroom. This book was written to help newly diagnosed children know they are not alone in this diagnosis and they can be successful in the classroom and in life with a little help.

www.ingramcontent.com/pod-product-compliance
Lightning Source LLC
Chambersburg PA
CBHW040317010626
45792CB00023B/1004